Dedicated

A wonderful mother and pe.　　　　　　　*.nuch*
and have never said than.　　　　*.nough.*
I love you more than .　　*.un say.*

Benjamin Peel

NOT A GAME FOR GIRLS

OBERON BOOKS
LONDON

WWW.OBERONBOOKS.COM

First published in 2018 by Oberon Books Ltd
521 Caledonian Road, London N7 9RH
Tel: +44 (0.) 20 7607 3637 / Fax: +44 (0.) 20 7607 3629
e-mail: info@oberonbooks.com
www.oberonbooks.com

PB ISBN: 9781786826497
E ISBN: 9781786826169

Cover image by Roger Pattison

Printed and bound by 4EDGE Limited, Hockley, Essex, UK.
eBook conversion by Lapiz Digital Services, India.

Visit www.oberonbooks.com to read more about all our books and to buy them. You
will also find features, author interviews and news of any author events, and you can
sign up for e-newsletters so that you're always first to hear about our new releases.

Printed on FSC accredited paper

10 9 8 7 6 5 4 3 2 1

Thanks

Not a Game for Girls has received much development help along the way with a rehearsed reading at The Space on the Isle of Dogs in 2013, and a shortened adapted version being performed as part of the BBC's WW1 at Home Event in Manchester in 2014. There are too many people to mention but I am thankful to all of them for their kind support.

I cannot thank Alison Young and Matthew Wignall enough at Off the Rock Productions in York for taking a punt on an unknown debut play by an unknown writer and turning it into a piece of theatre that surpassed my imaginings for which I will always be eternally grateful. Many thanks also to Jules Tipton for pitching it to Guildford School of Acting, inviting me to be part of the rehearsal process and directing a second production which showed wonderfully that the script is open to being staged in rather different ways. The cast and crew of both productions were equally fantastically supportive and instrumental in bringing it to life.

Now with its publication I am indebted to James Hogan and Oberon Books for their support of both the play and myself.

Most of all I would like to extend my profound appreciation to my parents for their continual encouragement and belief in my writing endeavours.

Foreword

I first became aware of the Dick, Kerr's Ladies in 2011 when the Women's World Cup was played. I was instantly hooked as I had no idea that women's football went that far back and indeed it started before then in the late nineteenth century.

After mulling over the idea of dramatising it for a while (I initially wrote a screenplay but converted it to a stage version rewriting it radically in the process) I began to do some internet research. I quickly realised that I would need to do more than that and read a few general history books about the period, plus some on both the team and the narrative of women's football.

This included Tim Tate's comprehensive *Girls with Balls: The Secret History of Women's Football* (John Blake Publishing, 2013) which documents the early beginnings of the women's game along with the social changes occurring simultaneously. I discovered that two of the best known players from those early days were Alice Woods and Lily Parr.

Alice and Lily were not part of the initial team assembled by Alfred Frankland but joined later. They both hailed from different parts of working class St Helens and, like the others in the side, saw in football the opportunity to escape from the strictures of a male-dominated society albeit for different reasons.

Although the play is based on real life characters and events I have in the name of dramatic licence not stuck to an exact historical timeline and have moved some episodes around and into my time frame. As it is impossible to relate the background of all eleven players from that very first side, I have created some fictional and some composite characters. It is of course anyway my own invented theatrical rendering of the Dick, Kerr's Ladies story up until a certain point in time that I felt to be a natural stopping point for the play.

However I hope that I have captured some of the spirit and camaraderie that led those women to ignore and defy the prevailing social attitudes from both genders and prove most emphatically that they were wrong to dismiss football as *Not a Game for Girls*.

Production History

Not a Game for Girls was first performed by Off the Rock Productions at Friargate Theatre, York, in June 2017 with the following cast and creative team:

ALICE WOODS	Hannah Jade Robbins
FLORRIE REDFORD	Kirsty Edwards
BETTY WILLIAMS	Sonia Di Lorenzo
JESSIE WALMSLEY	Georgie Smith
JACK HOLMES	Matthew Wignall
ALFRED FRANKLAND	Keir Brown
LILY PARR	Laura Castle
SOLDIER	Edie Palmer
MRS PARR	Samantha Hindman
MRS WOODS	Victoria Delaney
LEN WILLIAMS	Richard Thirlwall
MADELAINE OURRY	Natalie-Clare Brimicombe
HERBERT STANLEY	Guy Matthews
FOOTBALLERS ON FILM	Bronte Hobson, Riyadh Johnson, Becky Sheard and Tasha Stacey

Director	Alison Young
Assistant Director	Mike Hickman
Sound Design	Alexander King
Set Design	Paul Mason
Music Director	Samantha Hindman
Stage Manager	Ann Crossley
Assistant Stage Manager	Matt Pattison
Lighting	Harriet Mayne
Costume	Carly Brown
Producer	Matthew Wignall
Photography	Hannah Argyle
Film Footage and Trailers	Blue Tomato Studio
Catering	Michelle Gracias

Not a Game for Girls was subsequently performed by second year students at Guildford School of Acting in March 2018 with the following cast and creative team:

FLORRIE REDFORD	Sophie Abbott
LEN WILLIAMS/FRED/ DOCTOR/THE MINISTER	James Bibby
LILY PARR	Emma Brown
JACK HOLMES	Nathan Collins
MRS WOODS/PUB SINGER	Ishbel Cumming
ALFRED FRANKLAND	Reece Evans
MRS PARR/MADELAINE OURRY	Ellen Kretschmer
HERBERT STANLEY/ MATCH OFFICIAL	Rishi Manuel
ALICE WOODS	Laura Molyneux
JESSIE WALMSLEY	Ronay Poole
BETTY WILLIAMS/ WOMAN IN CHURCH	Brenna Simpson

All other roles played by members of the cast.

Director	Jules Tipton
Lighting	Laurie Bailey*
Sound Design	Daisy Edmonds*
Set/Costume Design	Ellie Brereton*
Voice Coach	Barbara Ward
Movement Director	Laura Weston
Production Manager	Roger Ness
Stage Manager	Claire Wilmore
Deputy Stage Manager	Samantha Kerrison
Assistant Stage Manager	Ellie Gregson*
Studio Manager	Dan Marsh
Scenic Construction	Jamie Fitzgerald
Production Electricians	Zachariah North/Oli Hancock
Lighting Programmer/ Operator	Dan Marsh
Wardrobe Supervisor	Vicki Halliday

Characters

ALFRED FRANKLAND
Manager at Dick, Kerr's manufacturers and team manager

JACK HOLMES
Ex-professional footballer

HERBERT STANLEY
Alfred Frankland's assistant

FLORRIE REDFORD
Captain of Dick, Kerr's team and centre forward

LILY PARR
Outside left

ALICE STANLEY NÉE WOODS
Centre half

JESSIE WALMSLEY
Defender

BETTY WILLIAMS
Goalkeeper

DAISY WALKER
Team member

MADELAINE OURRY
French goalkeeper

MRS WOODS

MRS PARR

LEN WILLIAMS

FRED

MINISTER

WOMAN IN CHURCH

Possible cast breakdown for eleven actors:

Actor 1 – Florrie Redford
Actor 2 – Jessie Walmsley/Daisy
Actor 3 – Betty Williams/Woman in church
Actor 4 – Lily Parr
Actor 5 – Alice Stanley née Woods
Actor 6 – Mrs Woods/Pub singer
Actor 7 – Mrs Parr/Madelaine Ourry
Actor 8 – Len Williams/Doctor Fred/The Minister
Actor 9 – Jack Holmes
Actor 10 – Alfred Frankland
Actor 11 – Herbert Stanley/FA official
(Referee who chalks scored etc.)

Production note

Settings and stage directions can be adapted and amended to
suit each individual playing space.

Acts/scenes

The play is in two acts and set between 1917-1921.
Half-time occurs between the acts.

Notes to the Players:

The movement sequences, including the football matches, were devised by the company developing ideas used in the original York production and are dependent on which actors/characters are available at that particular point in the play. For example, Betty Williams in goal until she leaves the team and Madelaine Ourry in goal when they play France. How the games are staged will also depend on whether the play is performed in traverse or not. If it is, the goal area for every game can be at the 'domestic' end although that it is up to each individual production.

The sequences on pages 48 and 56 respectively have additional commentary which reflects the Dick, Kerr's Ladies achievements, this can be recorded as part of the production sound design.

Many of the scenes flow into each other through the acting space with changes in location/shifts in time being marked through lighting design.

The author kindly acknowledges the contributions to the development of the script made by the York cast and their director, Alison Young of Off the Rock Productions, and the Guildford School of Acting cast and their director, Jules Tipton.

ACT I

PRELUDE

A bare open stage with the minimum of set. Depending on the space, it is preferred that the play is performed in traverse with a pitch marked out on the stage and scene settings indicated with furniture etc.

Alternatively if traverse is not possible projections on the back wall can also be used, as well as furniture to depict the setting, to display who the matches are between, the scores, half-time etc., and an on stage changing hut could be part of the set.

At one end are factory doors that open outwards with a street lamp to the side of them and a chalkboard to the other. The other end is the domestic.

Music of the 1920s plays as the audience enter.

LILY PARR, FLORRIE REDFORD, JESSIE WALMSLEY, BETTY WILLIAMS and MADELAINE OURRY are dressed in their Dick, Kerr's Ladies kit (black and white jerseys, blue shorts and a black and white striped hat) warming up, engaging in pre-match chat alongside their physical exercises: passing the leather football over their heads, under their legs, leap-frog, shadow boxing, gentle jogging, skipping.

As the music changes to something from 1978 with football crowd noise/ distorted white noise, the action freezes.

SCENE ONE

As the music shifts through the decades, the girls exit through the nearest exit in the space – except for LILY PARR. Three men in dark overcoats enter. One is carrying a head and shoulders portrait of a woman. The other two carry an easel.

They place the easel in front of the factory doors and stand aside.

LILY watches the men setting up the easel with her portrait on it, giving her name and dates: Lily Parr 1905-1978. LILY goes to stand next to it. Alternatively this could be done via a projection of a photograph of LILY PARR.

The men move to their opening position.

Football crowd/chanting sounds fade. LILY exits factory end as the rest of the mourners enter. 'Abide with Me' is sung as they reach their positions.

ALICE (now ALICE STANLEY, and elderly) moves to the centre spot.

ALICE: Lily, I well remember the first time I met you! You were a rough diamond all right, to say you were unconventional is an understatement. You were exasperating and infuriating but you were a great person to have on your side, both on and off the field. Woe betide any girl who had a pigtail though and it didn't matter if she played on the same side as you. You even had the dubious honour of being the first woman ever to be sent off for fighting on the pitch!

Eh, Lily, where did the time go?

Sfx of a noisy factory and an extract of a popular WW1 song.

ALICE exits. The mourners now become munitions factory workers.

Sfx of a noisy munitions factory fades up. Sfx of factory hooter.

SCENE TWO

FLORRIE, JESSIE and BETTY enter from the factory into the yard. FLORRIE has a football.

FLORRIE: Right then ladies, let's show these men they're talking rubbish.

BETTY: Think we'd better get back t'work soon.

JESSIE: What did Pop say, Florrie? Is he going to make you pay for t'broken window?

2

FLORRIE: No, he wants me to see if I can get a team together. Are you two interested?

JESSIE: I am. Who are we going to play?

FLORRIE: Other factory and munitions workers.

JESSIE: We'll show these men eh? We're just as good as 'em here and…

FLORRIE: What about you Betty?

BETTY: I don't know.

JESSIE: Come on, it'll be fun.

FLORRIE: I'm sure Len wouldn't want you moping about at home.

BETTY: I'll have a think on it.

The girls freeze in position as the focus shifts as JACK and ALFRED enter.

SCENE THREE

JACK (with a pronounced limp) and ALFRED (a well-dressed man in a three piece suit, fob watch, winter coat, bowler hat etc.).

JACK: You really think you can do this?

ALFRED: The ladies need a distraction from work and their men being away at the front. We all do.

JACK: I'm not sure this will work though, Mr Frankland.

ALFRED: If they're motivated they're more productive. The public need a distraction too.

JACK: There'll be a lot of doomsayers.

ALFRED: You're not wrong there. Well I'll show them that women can play football.

JACK: I hope you're right.

ALFRED: Aye, well, if I can't do my bit over there, I'll make sure I'm doing all I can here.

JACK: No one's thought of playing a game in a stadium before.

ALFRED: We'll raise more for the charities this way.

JACK: It's a hell of a lot of money you're asking for upfront though

ALFRED: These ladies'll fill Deepdale all right, you mark my words.

JACK: I hope you're right. The FA can be very bloody-minded in my experience.

ALFRED: Aye, well you should be grateful I've given you the benefit of the doubt and taken you on then.

JACK: They dropped that match fixing allegation against me you know: no evidence. Everyone else was at it though. But mud sticks.

ALFRED: I know Jack and I also know that you'll never be allowed near the men's game again.

JACK: And now I'm reduced to training a load of lasses. I'll be a laughing stock!

SCENE FOUR

JACK and ALFRED walk over to the ladies.

FLORRIE: Here, Betty – catch!

FLORRIE throws a ball at BETTY who tries to catch it but drops it.

Come on, Betty. I'm hoping you can be our goalkeeper.

JACK blows a whistle and the ladies gather together.

ALFRED: Right then, ladies. As you know. The Dick, Kerr's board have agreed that we can form a factory team and I'm to be your manager. Now, we haven't got much time before our first game on Christmas Day.

JESSIE: You're not wrong there.

ALFRED: Yes, thank you, Jessie. Now, you all know me – I am fair but firm. I expect nothing but the best from you. You will be impeccably turned out whether you are in your kit, or before and after a match. You will be punctual and show discipline at all times.

JESSIE: That might be a problem for Betty.

FLORRIE: Shut up, Jessie.

ALFRED: Yes, do be quiet now. I will only tolerate so much backchat and I wouldn't push it. Anyway, Florrie's your captain so I'd start listening to her sharpish.

JESSIE mutters an apology.

(*Beat.*) You're going to come in for quite a bit of stick, and we need to show we are serious both on and off the field, so I've brought in some help. This is Jack Holmes. I don't need to tell you about his illustrious time with Preston.

JACK: I did play for some other teams.

ALFRED: Let's forget about that shall we? He's going to help improve your skills in a few areas.

ALFRED exits.

JACK: I've got plenty of training ideas for you. Right let's see where we are.

JACK shouts instructions as they practice exercises for stamina and skill. They make various comments. The physical football is there but an imaginary ball is used for heading practice. They are all in the centre after JESSIE misses a header.

You're doing alright, but one thing you're all too scared of doing is heading the ball which is a crucial skill.

Right, you're going to take it turns to practice some headers.

Heading practice continues. JESSIE has a go and misses. The imaginary ball is thrown back and FLORRIE steps up.

That's *(slight beat)* good. Right, then, Florrie isn't it?

JACK throws an imaginary ball towards FLORRIE who misses it.

Don't be afraid. It'll hurt a little but not that much.

FLORRIE: I'm not scared.

JACK throws the imaginary ball again and FLORRIE forcefully heads it back.

JACK: That's good Florrie. A bit of aggression at last. Keep it up and you might just about be ready for the match on Christmas Day!

The ladies exit into the on stage hut or off stage to get changed.

ALFRED enters.

SCENE FIVE

The chalkboard is set up by the referee. He chalks on 'deepdale' and Dick, Kerr's Ladies vs Arundel Coulthard.

A brass band can be heard playing christmas carols. Sfx: crowd noise.

ALFRED: Merry Christmas, Jack.

JACK: Aye, and to you.

ALFRED: Is that drink I can smell on you?

JACK: Got to have a nip of something to keep out the cold, haven't I?

ALFRED: As long as was only a nip!

They take in the stadium and the crowd.

Have I done the right thing by asking you to train these ladies Jack?

JACK: How do you mean?

ALFRED: I need someone with enthusiasm to galvanise them. They're all nervous enough as it is.

JACK: You approached me.

ALFRED: Aye as I thought it was never right what they did to you. Be that as it may I need total commitment and loyalty from you Jack.

JACK: Aye and you'll get it. When those girls walk out onto the pitch that's all the encouragement they'll need. I can't describe the feeling Mr Frankland, Alf, and what I wouldn't give to have it again. They're ready for this.

ALFRED: But is everyone else?

The girls come out of the changing room in their kit. ALFRED addresses his team.

ALFRED: Well, I reckon we'll have raised near on two hundred pounds from this game. I know we've not had long to train for it but there's near ten thousand folk out here all come to see you play so just remember everything we've taught you and enjoy it.

A stylised game begins without a ball. The girls move for count of eight and freeze for count of eight. Pulsating music such as 'Dies Irae' from Karl Jenkins' 'Requiem' accompanies this and the other games. The half-time finishes on a freeze frame. ALFRED and JACK shout encouragement and instructions from the sidelines.

Sfx: whistle.

The ladies troop over to where ALFRED and JACK are.

JACK: This is embarrassing. We're a laughing stock. You can't have forgotten everything already.

ALFRED: They're just a bit nervous and the crowd don't know what to make of it.

FLORRIE: We've completely lost our shape.

BETTY: We're lucky they haven't scored yet.

FLORRIE: You just keep giving the ball away. I'm not getting any of it.

JESSIE: I'm not giving it away but I can't defend everything by myself.

FLORRIE: You need to listen to what I'm telling you and get the ball up to me.

JESSIE: I'm too busy clearing our lines.

BETTY: You could come back and help us.

FLORRIE: Then how do we attack them?

JACK: All right ladies. There's just too many silly mistakes being made.

ALFRED: You were getting better by the end of that half but you need to forget about the crowd watching you.

JACK: Or we'll be finished before we've even started.

ALFRED: You can do this and show them that women can play football.

Sfx: whistle.

The ladies go back onto the pitch.

FLORRIE: Come on, girls. We can do better than this. Concentrate.

Similar movement and freeze arrangement as before. JESSIE makes a crunching tackle.

ALFRED and JACK continue to shout encouragement and instructions.

The mounting scores are recorded using the chalkboard or the final score is projected at the end. The Dick Kerr's win four, nil.

Sfx: whistle/cheering and applause from crowd.

ALFRED and JACK – post-match chat with the team.

What did you think?

JACK: We were bloody lucky. Four nil flattered us.

ALFRED: You're not wrong. You're not bad and you could be good with a lot more training.

JACK: Are we really doing the right thing here?

JESSIE: How do you mean?

JACK: Playing women's football matches.

FLORRIE: Why shouldn't we?

JACK: I'm just not sure owt good can come of it.

ALFRED: We're raising money for the local hospital. *(Beat.)* I want this to be the best team in the country.

JACK: You need some better players then.

JACK and ALFRED exit and the team exit into the changing hut or off stage. The chalkboard is rubbed out and 'St Helens' is written on it.

SCENE SEVEN

LILY and ALICE enter in St Helen's football kit (black shorts and blue tops). They are practising dribbling and tackling. LILY barges into ALICE and knocks her flying.

LILY: Get up you bloody silly bugger. I was nowhere near you! Come on, Alice, get up.

ALICE: Let me get my breath back, Lily. I told you – a referee in a proper game won't let you get away with that.

LILY: I didn't bleeding do owt.

ALICE: And don't let him hear you swearing like that either.

LILY: It were me brothers who taught me how to cuss and spit.

ALICE: Yes, but referees don't like it.

LILY: Aye, my brothers said to do all that when his back's turned.

ALICE: What else did they say?

LILY: They said you've got the balls right enough, sis. You just need to learn a few tricks is all.

ALICE: Like what?

LILY: Look one way and kick the ball in t'other. Come on, let's practise some penalties.

ALICE: Not likely, not after last time. You nearly broke my hand.

LILY: Big bloody Jessie, you are!

ALICE: I think you'd be better off playing rugby.

LILY: There ain't any women's rugby teams.

A beat.

ALICE: I wish my brother was here.

LILY: Learning you all about the rules of the game? What was it you said to him?

ALICE: I said 'I may be a girl John but I can understand the offside rule.' I can't bear to think what it must be like over there. He never talks about it when he comes back.

LILY: Aye, it must be hard.

ALICE, still thinking about her brother, slowly moves into reverie. LILY regards her curiously.

ALICE: Fear no more the heat o' the sun,
    Nor the furious winter's rages;
    Thou thy worldly task hast done,
    Home art gone, and ta'en thy wages:
    Golden lads and girls all must,
    As chimney-sweepers, come to dust.

LILY: That sounds cheerful, Alice.

ALICE: I'm sorry. It's just that I know there's more going on than what we read in the papers.

LILY: I don't have time to read 'em. I best be getting home soon. Everyone else has gone.

ALICE: Come on let's have a quick run first. I'll give you a head start.

LILY: You'll still beat me.

LILY runs off stage and is followed by ALICE.

A recording of 'I Didn't Raise My Boy to Be a Soldier' is played as MRS WOODS and MRS PARR are each visited by a soldier. In MRS WOODS' case the soldier is her son who she lovingly embraces. While the other soldier hands MRS PARR a telegram.

The two soldiers and LEN WILLIAMS (married to BETTY WILLIAMS) sing a verse of 'When This Lousy War Is Over'.

The two soldiers drunkenly begin singing. LEN WILLIAMS, takes out his hip flask. Other cast members sing from off stage.

SOLDIERS: Oh, Mademoiselle from Armentieres,
Parlez-vous
Oh, Mademoiselle from Armentieres,
Parlez-vous
You didn't have to know her long,
To know the reason men go wrong!
Hinky-dinky, parlez-vous?

Oh, Mademoiselle from Armentieres,
Parlez-vous
Oh, Mademoiselle from Armentieres,
Parlez-vous
She's the hardest working girl in town,
But she makes her living upside down!
Hinky-dinky, parlez-vous?

(Shouting.) Come on, Len, your turn!!

LEN sings the final verse alone in an increasingly faltering voice.

Oh, Mademoiselle from Armentieres,
Parlez-vous

Oh, Mademoiselle from Armentieres,
Parlez-vous
She'll do it for wine, she'll do it for rum,
And sometimes for chocolate or chewing gum!
Hinky-dinky, parlez-vous?

The soldiers exit off stage. BETTY comes on and leads him away.

SCENE EIGHT

ALFRED gives a speech to the munitions factory workers (FLORRIE, JESSIE and BETTY) but it is also addressed out to the audience.

ALFRED: So, ladies and gentlemen, I can't put it any better than they said in the papers: 'History has seen a no more glorious day than the end of the Great World War, and the triumph of Great Britain and her Allies'.

Mr Dick and Mr Kerr would like me to extend their thanks to you all for the hard work and effort you have contributed here on the home front! It is thanks to your sterling efforts that our lads were able to continue the bombardments. Three million shells you have helped our factory produce during your time here in Preston.

However, I have been asked to warn you that – as you would expect – when the men return they will need jobs, and we will need to make room for them by, sadly, asking some you to step aside to make way for them.

FLORRIE: But that's not fair.

JESSIE: We worked just as hard as the men and got paid less.

ALFRED: Come on, ladies – you knew that this was always going to happen. The munition factories on the orders of the government are being disbanded and we're going back to making what we did before. Now, there'll be a notice by the door on your way out. If your name is on it then

I'm very sorry but we will be letting you go. Can the Dick, Kerr's Ladies come over to me please?

FLORRIE, JESSIE and BETTY go over to ALFRED as everyone else leaves.

I thought I would let you know personally that some names have been drawn at random and I'm sorry to say that both Florrie and Jessie that yours came out. Betty, you'll be kept on for the time being.

BETTY: Thank you. Might there be something for Len?

ALFRED: Maybe, when the time's right.

BETTY: Thank you.

BETTY leaves.

ALFRED: You knew it was always the case most of you would be let go once the men started arriving back.

FLORRIE: It still doesn't seem fair though.

JESSIE: Can we still play for the team if we're not working here though?

ALFRED: Certainly – we'll keep the team going, and Florrie will still be the captain.

FLORRIE: Do we still get our expenses?

ALFRED: Ten shillings a match, same as before. Now go on. I'll see you at practice.

ALFRED exits.

FLORRIE: I don't see why they're letting us go. We worked just as hard as the men, if not harder.

JESSIE: But we knew it would be over sometime. It seems funny doesn't it – us working in a factory, making shells, and playing football. George's mother is still giving me grief about playing.

FLORRIE: She's not, is she?

JESSIE: She reckons George won't be best pleased to see me cavorting about in shorts.

FLORRIE: I thought he knew.

JESSIE: He does, but he's too scared to say anything to his Mam.

FLORRIE: She reckons ladies wearing trousers is bad enough. She'll want things to go back to how they were before.

JESSIE: Not all of them surely? They can't!

FLORRIE: George'll want you at home when you're married.

JESSIE: George might have to think again.

JESSIE and FLORRIE exit.

SCENE NINE

LEN and BETTY WILLIAMS at home. LEN is seated at a table. BETTY is bringing the tea things in on a tray. The mugs and cutlery rattle as she carries them. LEN is obviously a bit drunk.

LEN: Do you have to make so much noise, woman?

BETTY: Sorry, I was getting us some tea…

Len, now the war's over Mr Frankland was saying that there will be more jobs for the boys, now they're coming back. Some of us have been let go to make room. Maybe I could ask Mr Frankland if there's a job for you there if you feel ready that is.

LEN: Betty I can't…

BETTY: No…course not… I had thought about training as a nurse…like Florrie wants to – Florrie from the factory – she plays football… It was only an idea…

LEN: A nurse?

BETTY: A silly idea… But I thought it might be a way I could help… The Whittingham is doing good work helping men, like you, who are not injured as such but are still troubled…you know, troubled by what they saw and –

LEN: The Whittingham's a mental hospital.

BETTY: Well, it's doing good things – and we're helping by raising money for it with the football matches.

LEN: I don't need help! I told you, your place is here, with me – not going off playing football.

BETTY: You don't know what the football means to me, Len. To all of us. If you just came and saw us play.

LEN: Is our tea ready yet?

There is a knock at the door. LEN is startled. He drinks from his hip flask as BETTY exits. She enters with ALFRED.

ALFRED: I'm very sorry to trouble you, Mr Williams, but I've just called round to see if you'd reconsider letting Betty play for the team. She really enjoys it and…

LEN: Football's not a game for lassies to be playing and I'm surprised you encourage it.

ALFRED: It was the government that encouraged it.

LEN: Aye well, the war's over now and I didn't fight it only to come back and see my missus running about a field making a fool of herself.

ALFRED: Isn't it up to Betty?

LEN: What did you do in the war?

ALFRED: I don't see how that's pertinent.

LEN: Pertinent! You're bloody impertinent showing up on me
doorstep spouting nonsense. How in hell's name would
you know? The country's gone to the bleeding dogs.

ALFRED: All right. I'm sorry. I'll see myself out.

ALFRED exits off stage. LEN turns to BETTY.

LEN: Did you put him up to coming round here?

BETTY: No. But he's a good man.

LEN: And I'm not?

BETTY: I didn't mean – of course you are. But I can see
you're different since you came back. I know awful
things happened over there in France. But you don't say
anything about it.

LEN: You wouldn't want to know.

BETTY: I want to help you. Getting drunk won't help though.

LEN: It helps me forget. For a while at least. *(Beat.)* You don't
want to give up playing football do you?

BETTY: No, but I will.

LEN: I don't understand you or any of this anymore. I'm
going out.

BETTY: Stay here please Len and talk to me. It doesn't have
to be about the war.

LEN exits and BETTY waits then exits too.

*The cast sing the first verse of 'I Vow to Thee, My Country'
unaccompanied.*

17

SCENE 10

Sfx: game being played/crowd noise.

ALFRED enters. LILY (in civvies) runs past ALFRED with a ball in her hands. ALFRED tries to stop her but she runs past him. She is followed onto the stage by ALICE. ALFRED manages to stop her.

ALFRED: That was a fine game you played, young lady.
I would like to ask if you'd consider playing for Dick,
Kerr's. We'll pay you ten shillings a match and the
charabanc could collect you in St Helens. By the way
I'd be very grateful if you could extend my offer to your
outside left. Miss Parr, isn't it? Here's my card.

ALFRED tips his hat and exits. ALICE is left there, calling after him.

ALICE: I'll try my best sir but she's a law to herself is Lily Parr.
I'm not even sure where she lives.

SCENE ELEVEN

Sfx: atmospheric pub piano, singing, drinking noises to establish neighbourhood.

ALICE walks through a dark and foggy street. A sudden blaring of drunken song from a pub can be heard. This makes her nervous but she continues looking for LILY's house along the street.

ALICE: Lily? Lily?

LILY enters dribbling a ball.

LILY: What do you bloody want Woods?

ALICE: Dick, Kerr's wants us to play for them Lily.

LILY: What really?

ALICE: Yes, really. This is where you live?

LILY: Yes, it is. Why?

ALICE: I've never been to this part of town before.

LILY: I can believe that.

ALICE: Do you think your mother will let you play for Dick, Kerr's?

LILY: She'll say if you look out for us then I can, though I can take care of meself.

ALICE: I know.

LILY: Me mam don't get why I like sport, but me brothers do.

ALICE: My mother doesn't either.

LILY: Being good at summat is the only way to get noticed round here. Everyone just keeps their head down and does the same thing day in day out.

ALICE: I know what you mean.

LILY: Do you?

ALICE: People aren't so different. I'd better be getting back before mother starts to worry.

LILY: I'll walk some of the way with you.

Both ALICE and LILY enter their respective homes with LILY's being at the factory end. MRS PARR and MRS WOODS enter. MRS WOODS brings in a trophy. Furniture is set.

SCENE 12

MRS PARR is attending to the washing in a tin bath. LILY looks on.

LILY: But Mam, he's said I can get ten bob each time I play.

MRS PARR: If Alice is not going then you ain't neither. Her mam says she's needed where she is and Lord knows I could do wiv some help an' all.

ALFRED enters.

ALFRED: Hello? I was told to come through here. My name is Alfred Frankland.

MRS PARR: My, we didn't know you were coming, Mr Frankland.

ALFRED: Alfred, please. Didn't Lily tell you I would be?

MRS PARR: No, she didn't.

LILY: I wasn't sure he would.

ALFRED: I'm a man of my word. I've come to ask if you'll reconsider and let Lily play for Dick, Kerr's?

MRS PARR: Lily, go and see what the rest of 'em are up to. I want to hear what Mr Frankland has got to say without you opening your big gob.

LILY exits.

Now then, I'm listening.

ALFRED: Mrs Parr, without wanting to overstate the case, I believe your daughter to be the best player I've ever seen and essential to my plans. If you're agreeable I could lodge her with the family of another of my young players in Preston. We could find her a job at the factory so she'd have money to send home. I can't say any fairer than that.

MRS PARR: I'll think on it and let you know.

ALFRED: Thank you for your time.

ALFRED exits. LILY enters.

LILY: Well?

MRS PARR: Well I reckon you're old enough to make your own mind up and if it gets you away from all this…

LILY: I'll want me own room.

MRS PARR: You'll have to be grateful for what you're given and knuckle down to the job in case the football doesn't work out.

LILY: I heard what he said. He reckons I'm the greatest player he's ever seen.

MRS PARR: Well, don't let him down then. You've been given a chance to do summat wiv your life, Lily. It's more than most of us around here get. I love you girl, but Lord knows you can be hard work. Anyway, before you go all hoity-toity on us, the little'un needs changing and feeding.

LILY: I won't miss cleaning up his shite.

SCENE 13

Opposite end of the space: chair set.

MRS WOODS and ALICE enter the parlour domestic end of the set. MRS WOODS brings a trophy in with her. ALFRED enters.

MRS WOODS: My young Alice wandering about the streets of Gerards Bridge at night looking for this waif Lily Parr and all at your beckoning.

ALFRED: I'm very sorry about that but I didn't imagine that she'd go out like… Whose is that trophy?

MRS WOODS: Its Alice's, from when she won the eighty yard sprint.

ALFRED: She's a proper little rocket, and no mistake.

MRS WOODS: I'll not be budged, Mr Frankland. You can use as much fancy talk as you like. Alice is staying here where she's needed. My son John came back from the war, and I'm not losing another one.

ALICE: It's only Preston.

MRS WOODS glares at her.

ALFRED: Right, I'll tell you what I'll do. Alice can play for Dick, Kerr's but she won't have to work for them. She can stay here and just come and play for us. How does that sound?

MRS WOODS: I'll have a good ponder on it.

ALFRED exits.

ALICE: Please let me go Mother. Dick, Kerr's is the best ladies football team going.

MRS WOODS: I don't know what your poor father would think of you running about a football pitch.

ALICE: He'd have been proud of me.

MRS WOODS: I'd just about won the church around to the idea of your running but this playing football...well, they are not too happy about it at all. But you're right about your father. He always treated you the same as your brothers.

ALICE: I've been playing for St Helens for long enough. Anyway, not everyone at the church thinks the same way. It's only the silly old Minister.

MRS WOODS: Alice, don't talk about him like that.

ALICE: The nonsense he came out with during the war makes...sorry mother, but I agree with John.

MRS WOODS: All right. Stop mithering me. I said I'd think about and I will.

Benches are moved on in readiness for training.

The Dick, Kerr's Ladies are all getting ready for a training session. ALFRED, HERBERT and JACK enter. ALICE and LILY enter. They stand apart from the others, still in their st helens kit.

ALFRED: Good morning, ladies. I'd like to introduce you to some new people. First of all, this is Herbert Stanley, and he's going to be my assistant. And these two are Lily Parr and Alice Woods. I'm sure you remember them from when we played St Helens. Their skills will really strengthen the side. Right, over to you for the time being Jack please. I just need to speak to Herbert.

HERBERT and ALICE exchange coy looks. HERBERT exits with ALFRED.

LILY: Come on, Alice. Never mind him.

ALICE: I don't know what you mean.

LILY: I saw you looking at each other. He don't look like he's even started shaving yet.

JESSIE: Hey you, Parr.

LILY: What?

JESSIE: You'd better not try and pull my hair again or I swear I'll swing for you.

LILY: Like to see you try.

FLORRIE: What's going on over here?

ALICE: Nothing. Is there, Lily?

LILY: No.

JACK: If you lot have finished gossiping then perhaps we can start. I want you to pair up and practice some dribbling and tackling.

The ladies pair up and begin the practice. LILY is with FLORRIE. FLORRIE tries to dribble around her but LILY goes in with a hard tackle that leaves FLORRIE writhing on the ground. LILY is surrounded by the other players.

JESSIE: What the hell was that?

LILY: I just tackled her. Not my fault she didn't get out of the road.

JACK: It's meant to be a practice session. Someone help Florrie to the bench.

JESSIE: You're an idiot, Lily. You've most likely injured her.

FLORRIE: What do you expect from someone who comes from Gerards Bridge?

LILY: You'd better watch what you're saying.

JESSIE: Or what?

FLORRIE: Come on Jessie. Just ignore her.

JESSIE, LILY and FLORRIE exit. ALFRED enters.

ALFRED: What just happened there?

JACK: Your new signing just took a lump out of Florrie.

ALFRED: She's a strong girl, alright.

JACK: Aye, but is that all she's got?

ALFRED: She's a raw talent I know, but I think she's got what it takes to be truly great. I'm sure you can bring that out of her.

JACK: I'm not sure I share your confidence.

ALFRED: I know I'm right.

JACK: Aye, I expect you think you are.

ALFRED: I don't expect backchat from you.

JACK: Well, if you wanted a back room 'yes man', you should have looked elsewhere. Not that you'd have found many ex-pros to help you out.

ALFRED: I'm sorry, Jack. She could be great but I just hope I haven't unbalanced the team.

ALFRED and JACK exit.

SCENE FIFTEEN

FLORRIE and JESSIE enter and sit on the bench. FLORRIE is nursing her injury. JESSIE paces.

JESSIE: Why don't they understand how much I love playing? I don't know why people are so prim and proper about it.

FLORRIE: So, tell me exactly what's been said

JESSIE: George's mother told me – in no uncertain terms – that it's not a game for girls.

FLORRIE: Have they ever come to see you play?

JESSIE: Don't be daft!

FLORRIE: What does George say?

JESSIE: He just wants things to be how they were before. All we seem to do is argue all the time.

FLORRIE: It's difficult for them.

JESSIE: He's been different ever since he got back… It's like I'm getting to know him all over again. I know terrible things happened over there.

FLORRIE: Things have changed for all of us. Our men have got the vote now.

JESSIE: Yes, and I just want to go on playing football, it's important to me but he can't seem to understand that.

FLORRIE: He's had a rough time.

JESSIE: I know that, but it wasn't easy for us either. Playing football was…an escape I guess.

FLORRIE: It still is.

JESSIE: We can forget everything for a bit. He says he'll never forget though.

FLORRIE: What will you do?

JESSIE: I don't know. It feels like we're at a crossroads. I've given him the engagement ring back.

FLORRIE: How did he take that?

JESSIE: Better than I thought.

FLORRIE: What about his mother?

JESSIE: He hasn't told her yet.

FLORRIE: There'll be fireworks when she finds out.

JESSIE: Aye there will.

SCENE SIXTEEN

Furniture set up.

Benches stacked to form the bar.

The lights come up on the ladies in a pub. FLORRIE, JESSIE and BETTY make their way over to the chairs. FLORRIE and JESSIE are given coats to put on over their kit and take off their hats all whilst the song continues.

SINGER: On a cold December morning
    He went into the ground
    On a cold December morning
    My laddie was Hell forth bound

    In hell hot mines as black as pitch
    The coal dust choked them all
    With a rumble deep as thunder
    The crumbling passage falls
    The brave men trapped inside
    Final thoughts of a family's pride

LEN enters and stands apart from everyone.

    On a cold December morning
    He went down into the ground
    On that cold December morning
    My laddie was heaven bound

Sung to the tune of 'His Eye Is On The Sparrow'

(https://www.youtube.com/watch?v=_95X3rzRJ1w#)

FLORRIE: How is everything, Betty?

BETTY: Sometimes something happens and I see flashes of the old Len. Every time I try and talk to him though he just clams up.

JESSIE: He was so carefree and gentle before.

BETTY: I can't bear to see him like this. Sometimes he wakes up screaming and then I have to comfort him like a child.

FLORRIE: Shell shock they call it don't they? Can you not get him some help Betty?

BETTY: It's not just my Len, though, is it?

LEN: How long are you going to be here for?

27

BETTY: Not long. I thought you were at home?

LEN: I was, but I thought you'd be back soon.

BETTY: I just wanted a quick drink after work.

LEN: What are all you women doing in a pub, any road?

FLORRIE: Things have changed, Len.

LEN: Don't I bloody know it. Come on, let's go home.

JESSIE: She'll go when she's ready, not when you say.

LEN: Who are you to tell me what to do?

JESSIE: I'm Betty's friend.

There is a loud off stage noise of a glass smashing. LEN throws himself to the ground and begins to cry and shake. BETTY goes to try and comfort him.

FLORRIE: Come on Jessie. Let's leave them to sort it out between them. Jessie.

FLORRIE and JESSIE exit.

BETTY: It's all right, Len.

LEN: Betty. It wasn't my fault... It wasn't –

BETTY: I know, love. Come on – let's get you home... I'll give up the football, but will you please try and get some help?

LEN: I don't need help.

BETTY: You do, my love.

LEN: No. I just need you.

BETTY: Come on. Let's go home. We can talk more there.

They exit.

SCENE SEVENTEEN

Furniture set domestic end. MRS WOODS is in the armchair, reading.

ALICE meets HERBERT on the doorstep of her house.

HERBERT: Will your mother like me? Do I look presentable?

ALICE: You look fine. Come in… Mother, this is Herbert.

HERBERT: Good afternoon, Mrs Woods. I'm very pleased to meet you.

MRS WOODS: The pleasure is all mine. *(Beat.)* Herbert. Do sit down.

ALICE: I'll just go and get my things.

She exits.

HERBERT: It's a lovely house you have here Mrs Woods. Very *(beat)* tasteful.

MRS WOODS: Cleanliness is next to godliness.

HERBERT: Of course… Yes, we won't be out too late, Mrs Woods, as I know Alice has a game tomorrow. I thought we could just go for a stroll as it's a fine evening and take tea somewhere.

An awkward beat.

MRS WOODS: Yes, very nice. Are you ready yet Alice?

ALICE enters.

ALICE: Yes, sorry to keep you waiting.

HERBERT: That's all right. Well, if you are ready? It was nice to meet you, Mrs Woods.

MRS WOODS: Yes, and you. Have a pleasant evening. And remember the good Lord is always watching.

MRS WOODS exits.

ALICE and HERBERT walk through a leafy park.

HERBERT: Thank you for coming out tonight, Alice.

ALICE: That's all right, although I can't stay out too long.

HERBERT: No, not the night before a match. I think you're very good at playing football, Alice. I like watching you.

ALICE: That's nice of you to say Herbert... Do you enjoy working for Pop... Mr Frankland, sorry?

HERBERT: I do, yes, but I don't think I'd get away with calling him Pop. It's interesting and full of different challenges.

ALICE: I bet it is, working with a ladie's football team.

They sit on a bench.

HERBERT: Did I make a good impression, on your mother?

ALICE: I'm sure she liked you.

HERBERT: So, she wouldn't mind us walking out?

ALICE: I wouldn't mind it either... It wouldn't bother you – courting someone who plays football?

HERBERT: Of course not.

ALICE: My mother gets a lot of snide comments from our church and so do I.

HERBERT: Are you religious then?

ALICE: Yes, but not as much as mother and I only go to please her really. *(Beat.)* Don't worry. I don't mind if you are not. John refused to go any more after he came back from the trenches.

HERBERT: I can understand that. I wasn't out there for long but it was long enough.

ALICE: You men won't talk about it much though. John won't.

HERBERT: It's something I would rather forget.

ALICE: Some of them, and especially the Minister are trying to pressure me to stop playing.

HERBERT: What? That's ridiculous. If it's something you enjoy why should you give it up?

ALICE: They don't think it's ladylike or godly. I don't know what to do.

HERBERT: Why not?

ALICE: It's tearing mother apart. Since father died the church is everything to her and her faith got even stronger when John came home. She feels like he's abandoned the church.

HERBERT: But you shouldn't have to sacrifice something that makes you happy. Lord knows there's been enough of that already. Come on, let's go and find that tea shop.

They exit.

SCENE EIGHTEEN

ALFRED and BETTY enter from the factory end.

BETTY: I can't play for the team and look after Len any more. It's just too much.

ALFRED: I'll be sorry to lose you. Good goalkeepers are hard to come by.

BETTY: I'm very sorry to be letting you down.

ALFRED: You're not letting anybody down, least of all me. I'm sure we can work something out.

BETTY: I need to put my husband first.

ALFRED: There's people out there who can help. The Salvation Army for one.

BETTY: I've finally managed to get him to see a doctor. He wants him to go into the Whittingham.

ALFRED: And will he?

BETTY: He thinks he'll be going into the loony bin.

ALFRED: They do some very good work there.

BETTY: Aye, I know.

ALFRED: You can always come back you know.

BETTY: I don't think I'll be doing that.

ALFRED: Is he no better at all?

BETTY: Some days are better than others, but he will never be my Len again. Thank you though for all that you've done.

ALFRED: You look after yourself now.

They exit.

SCENE NINETEEN

Match day – Liverpool.

The Dick, Kerr's Ladies enter in their kit and begin warming up for the game, putting their boots on etc.

JESSIE: How's the training going, Flo?

FLORRIE: Really well, thanks.

JESSIE: Better than the factory work was?

FLORRIE: Nursing's not a picnic.

JESSIE: Tiring?

FLORRIE nods at the massive understatement.

Surprised you've got the energy for this lark.

FLORRIE: *(Grinning.)* Wouldn't miss it for the world.

LILY enters still dressed in ordinary clothes.

LILY: Don't know about Dick, Kerr's Ladies, it looks like a bloody trip to Lourdes to me!

ALFRED enters accompanied by JACK and HERBERT.

ALFRED: You're late.

LILY: Sorry Pop.

ALFRED: You're not playing.

LILY: *(Exasperated.)* The tram broke down.

ALFRED: I don't care. You should leave enough time.

FLORRIE: We don't need her anyway.

LILY: What did you say?

FLORRIE: You heard me.

LILY: I'm the best player here and you know it.

ALFRED: Ladies…

JESSIE: Listen to her.

FLORRIE: Aye, she reckons she's better than us wanting a room all to herself.

ALFRED: Ladies…

LILY: What are youse on about? None of you would share with me anyway.

JESSIE: Too bloody right.

ALFRED: *(Shouting.)* Right that's enough. Pack it in.

Beat whilst the players calm down.

ALFRED: Right if you're all quite finished… I've got some news. I've arranged for the French national team to come over and play us over four games. And the last one…will be at Stamford Bridge.

ALICE: London!

FLORRIE: By eck!

JESSIE: I've never been further than Blackpool.

The team all troop out of the changing area. LILY puts her bag down and starts to remove her coat.

ALFRED: *(To LILY.)* Don't bother. You can sit with me on the bench.

JACK: You're not playing her! *(Clocks the look he gets.).* All right you're the boss.

LILY lights a cigarette as she makes her way to the on stage bench.

SCENE TWENTY

Football stand: game and crowd noise. Followed by whistle for full time. A football sequence plays out.

ALFRED, JACK and LILY are sitting on the bench. LILY smokes moodily whilst ALFRED and JACK animatedly move about. Score on chalkboard reads 'Liverpool 2 Dick, Kerr's Ladies 1'. Final whistle.

JACK, ALFRED and HERBERT exit – LILY exits in the opposite direction to them. ALICE, JESSIE and FLORRIE remain. ALICE puts a coat on over her football kit.

FLORRIE: That ref needs his eyes checking. That should have been a penalty.

JESSIE: You were in a bad mood the whole game though. Summat the matter?

FLORRIE: Bloody men. More trouble than they're worth.

JESSIE: Not all the time. Must be some good-looking doctors at the hospital.

FLORRIE: I spend all week being talked down to because they think nurses haven't got brains.

JESSIE: You can't be too choosy. It's not as if there's plenty of men to go around.

FLORRIE: All the more reason to be choosy then.

JESSIE: Wish someone would come and sweep me off me feet.

FLORRIE: He'd need to have some muscles!

JESSIE: Bugger off, you cheeky mare.

FLORRIE: I'd rather have a job and a bit of independence meself.

JESSIE: Oh yes, and how are you going to do that?

FLORRIE: Canada wants nurses.

JESSIE: You want to go to Canada?

FLORRIE: Why not? It's more forward-looking than this country.

JACK enters.

JACK: Has anyone seen the match ball?

ALICE: Has anyone seen Lily?

FLORRIE: She's disappeared.

JESSIE: There's your answer then.

JACK: The little minx. *(Beat.)* He should have played her today though.

They all exit.

SCENE TWENTY-ONE

LILY enters carrying a bag. Followed by ALICE.

ALICE: Why did you disappear after the game?

LILY: He didn't play me, did he?

ALICE: He's really disappointed in you, Lily. You're not making any friends either.

LILY: I'm not here to make friends – I'm here to play bloody football! And Pop should be disappointed, seeing as we didn't win.

ALICE: Don't swear like that Lily. It's not ladylike. He's taken a big chance on us and he's paying us a good wage.

LILY: And why's that? It's cos he needs us. At least that's what I overheard him telling me mam about me.

ALICE: No one's bigger than the team Lil.

LILY: Come on, he wanted us both to make the team better.

ALICE: Well, even if that's true it doesn't do to be late all the time and sulk when he doesn't play you. Oh, and run off with the ball after a game.

LILY subconciously shuffles the bag nearer to her with a foot.

LILY: I don't know what you mean.

ALICE: What is it you want, Lily?

LILY: I don't want to work in a factory for the rest of me life Alice. I want summat else. When I'm on the football pitch it's like… I dunno…like I'm somewhere else for an hour and a half.

ALICE: I know what you mean. It's like you are someone else as well. Just all us girls together.

They make some movements with an imaginary ball.

LILY: I'd be nowt without football. When I'm playing I can forget about everything else and just think about making a tackle or trying to score.

ALICE: It's a wonderful feeling being out there with so many people watching you. I've tried to explain it to mother but I can't seem to put how I feel into words which I usually can and then I get cross with myself really and…

LILY: Sometimes I think I'm different from other girls.

ALICE: I thought I was a bit of a tomboy until I met you but there's nothing wrong with that.

LILY: No, it's not that…it's I don't know. I think I like…

ALICE: What are you trying to say? I don't understand.

LILY: No, you're not listening Alice. You don't know me at all. You reckon you're better than me with your airs and graces. I know what you all think. There goes that thick silly Lily Parr. She'll never amount to owt. Well I don't need all this. I'll go back to St Helens.

LILY jumps up and runs out leaving her bag behind.

ALICE picks up the bag.

ALICE: Lily come back. I don't think that. You're an amazing footballer. Lily!

ALICE runs off after her.

SCENE TWENTY-TWO

The doors (factory end) are opened by the MINISTER as a church service has ended. MRS WOODS, accompanied by HERBERT, shakes his hand, followed by another WOMAN.

WOMAN: That was a lovely service Minister. It's wonderful to see so many people listening to the Lord's words – isn't it, Mrs Woods?

MRS WOODS: It certainly is.

WOMAN: Although we've not see your Alice here in recent weeks.

HERBERT: She's usually tired from a match on –

MRS WOODS: Thank you, Herbert!

WOMAN: Well, Minister, I'm a little surprised you've had nothing to say on the subject – I thought you disapproved of these ladie's football teams.

MINISTER: Well I do think that perhaps…

WOMAN: You told me that it's ungodly and unladylike.

MRS WOODS has overheard this.

MRS WOODS: They have raised thousands for charity, and wounded soldiers. How is that ungodly?

WOMAN: Seems you've bred a family of non-believers, Mrs Woods, your John's not shown his face either since he came home. It's a disgrace isn't it Minister?

MINISTER: 'Draw near to God, and he will draw near to you.' James, chapter four, verse eight.

WOMAN: And women showing their legs is an abomination in the sight of God. Something really must be done.

MRS WOODS: I wasn't happy about her playing football but I've seen what it means to her and what they've all achieved.

MINISTER: It lacks decorum and sense of propriety.

WOMAN: The war's over. There's no need for it any more.

MRS WOODS: You've always been a vindictive interfering busybody. You should keep your nasty opinions to yourself and your mouth shut.

MINISTER: Mrs Woods. Apologise at once – she does have a point!

MRS WOODS: I will not apologise! No one criticises me or my family!

HERBERT: I can't believe you just said that.

MRS WOODS: Well – who does she think she is? Narrow-minded, that's what I call it!

MINISTER: Everyone is free to express their views in my church, within reason, and if you don't like the way I run things, Mrs Woods, then it may be best if you found yourself another place of worship until your daughter decides to give up such an unsuitable sport!

The MINISTER and the WOMAN go back into the church and slam the doors. MRS WOODS exits.

ALICE enters. HERBERT meets her.

HERBERT: Alice! Thank goodness!

ALICE: What is it?

HERBERT: The Minister is threatening to throw your mother out of the church.

ALICE: What! why?

HERBERT: Someone was attacking you, and your mother stood up for you. The Minister sided with the other woman and he's saying your mother can't go back until she apologises and says you won't play football anymore. Come on Alice.

HERBERT exits, following MRS WOODS. ALICE opens LILY's bag and takes out the ball.

ALICE: What's so wrong about a group of ladies wanting to kick this about a field?

Sfx: whistle.

'Half-time' is chalked up onto the board.

End of Act 1.

ACT II

SCENE ONE

A church hall-type space. The welcome reception for the French team.

As the house lights fade down a song is sung whilst ALICE, HERBERT, FRED, MADELAINE, JESSIE and FLORRIE are on stage. The song is to the tune of 'After the Ball' arranged by David Wall.

SINGER: Mother she told me don't stay up late
It leads to moral decay
Well I've got news for you mater
It's too late to hear what you say

Life is too short, let's have some fun
Bright lights entice me in
I'll live my life like I'm on the run
For I don't believe in sin

Now I like to play so fast and fly
And go for a spin in those wheels
Buy me a drink, come on don't be shy
The night's young let's see what it reveals

Life is too short, let's have some fun
Bright lights entice me in
I'll live my life like I'm on the run
For I don't believe in sin

Mother she told me don't stay up late
It leads to moral decay
Well I've got news for you mater
It's too late to hear what you say

Mother she told me don't stay up late
It leads to moral decay
Well I've got news for you mater
Should have listened to you that day

Couples dance (including ladies together) to 'After the Ball' instrumental: a slow waltz. FRED and MADELAINE dance together, FRED's hand keeps slipping down but MADELAINE puts it back on her waist. ALICE and HERBERT dance as a couple.

Dialogue intersperses the singing and waltzing.

ALICE: I really don't know what I'm going to do.

HERBERT: Will you still want to carry on playing when we have a family?

ALICE: No, because I'll have them to look after.

HERBERT: Look, I know we're not that religious but it would please your mother if we went to church especially now that we're engaged.

ALICE: I don't want to give up sport altogether, you know.

HERBERT: I know you don't. You're not a bad tennis player. You sometimes beat me.

ALICE: Sometimes? I just hope we manage to get the Minister to agree we can get married there!

The music and dancing starts again. ALICE and HERBERT exit. The music stops and the dancers freeze in position. JACK and LILY enter.

JACK: Hey Lily, wait there a minute.

LILY: What do you want?

JACK: Straight to the point as always. *(Beat.)* You're a good player Lily but you could be great. *(Beat.)* You know you remind me of meself when I was your age.

LILY: How?

JACK: Full of anger and resentment.

LILY: You don't know me.

JACK: No, I don't but I know your background. Not much different to mine as it 'appens.

LILY: So.

JACK: So, Lily Parr, you can either let your resentment get the better of you or you can let your football do the talking. Think on.

Music starts and the couples dance as JACK exits and ALFRED enters. The music lowers and the dancers continue then freeze in position.

ALFRED: What can I do for you, Lily?

LILY: I'm worried about Alice, Pop.

ALFRED: She seems to be somewhere else at the moment.

LILY: Her mam's really under pressure from her church. They don't like Alice playing.

ALFRED: Thanks for letting me know.

LILY: Is everything all right, Pop?

ALFRED: I started this team as I thought that with the men away people could do with some football to watch.

LILY: And to raise money?

ALFRED: Yes, but the war finished and a lot of people reckoned that would be it. But I thought no, these women are getting something out of this so why not carry on.

LILY: And we are doing.

ALFRED: Yes we are but…oh never mind me, Lily.

There is an awkward beat.

LILY: I want to say sorry, Pop.

ALFRED: What for?

LILY: For being an idiot.

ALFRED: *(Laughs.)* Go on, you daft apeth.

The music starts again and the couples dance as ALFRED exits and LILY crosses to the Dick, Kerr's Ladies. The dancing and music continue. ALFRED sits at a table and is joined by ALICE who uncouples herself from HERBERT, who exits.

LILY: How much longer is this going to go on for? I'm so hungry I could eat a horse.

FLORRIE: Lily! Keep your voice down.

LILY: Why, that's what they eat int' it?

JESSIE: That's never their goalie. She'll be bloody lost between the posts.

FLORRIE: Lily don't eat like it's the last meal you'll ever see.

LILY: Shut up, Florrie.

FLORRIE: What were you talking to Pop about?

LILY: Nowt for you to know about.

FLORRIE: What's happened to Woods? Why is she not here?

JESSIE: I've heard she's not going to play for us anymore.

FLORRIE: What, why?

JESSIE: Her mam won't let her.

LILY: No, you've got it wrong.

JESSIE: What do you know about it then?

FLORRIE: Yes, come on tell.

LILY: I don't know owt, all right?

JESSIE: You know more than you're letting on.

LILY: Well, what if I do?

JESSIE: Come on let's leave her to stew.

FLORRIE: Do you not want to make friends, Lily?

LILY: Not with some of the likes of you?

JESSIE: Leave her, Florrie. She's in one of her funny moods
again.

*The dancing and music stops again and ALFRED is joined on one
part of the stage by ALICE.*

ALFRED: I've been speaking with Mr Routledge, your
Minister's boss. He said that he's had a bit of an argument
with that Minister of yours.

ALICE: What about?

ALFRED: Well the Minister thinks that it's unbecoming for
ladies to play football. Mr Routledge however thinks that
it's a good way for young ladies to expend their energies.
He also told me that your Minister is soon to retire.

ALICE: Is he? I didn't know that.

ALFRED: Politics is everywhere, Alice, even in religion.

ALICE: I didn't think a Minister could be as horrible as he's
been.

ALFRED: Men of the cloth are not infallible, Alice. Right, I
expect to see you in Blackpool.

ALICE: Are you a religious man, Pop?

ALFRED: Not really. I go, but that's only to please my wife. I don't think he'd object to ladies playing football though.

ALICE grimaces and clutches her stomach.

Are you all right?

ALICE: Yes, it's just a bit of tummy cramp.

ALFRED: It's not, you know, your time of…that is…your monthly…

ALICE: No, it's not that.

ALFRED: Well, if that does ever affect you I need to know but you should see a doctor about this.

ALICE: It's nothing. It's probably just something I ate.

Music starts and the couples dance again. ALICE joins the other Dick, Kerr's Ladies. The music and dancing continue and ALFRED is joined by MADELAINE OURRY who breaks away from FRED, who goes and sits near the Dick, Kerr's Ladies.

MADELAINE: It wasn't wrong what they told me.

ALFRED: What's that then?

MADELAINE: That the Lancashire girls are big and strong.

ALFRED: Oh aye. They're that all right, Mademoiselle…?

MADELAINE: Ourry. I do not think it wrong for women to play football. They are as graceful as ballet dancers. They do not play like men, they play fast but not vigorous football.

ALFRED: There's nothing wrong with my girl's vigour. I hope you have a good time and everyone behaves.

ALFRED goes to leave.

MADELAINE: You are not staying?

ALFRED: No it's not my cup of tea.

ALFRED exits. MADELAINE joins the Dick, Kerr's Ladies. LILY is moodily smoking.

JESSIE: You ready for us, then?

MADELAINE: You may have won the games so far but we are more, how do you say, elegant and not just playing football?

JESSIE: But not modest.

MADELAINE: Pardon?

FRED gets up and whispers something in ALICE WOOD's ear. ALICE pushes him away.

ALICE: That's disgusting. You ought to be ashamed of yourself. Just because I play football it don't mean that…

LILY: Get away from her, you dirty old sod.

FRED: It were only a joke. I know you all play football, but I didn't realise it was for the other side.

LILY raises her fist to him. FRED ducks and dives a bit. LILY advances on him again.

FRED: Bloody women.

FRED exits. MADELAINE puts her arm around LILY.

MADELAINE: Lily, don't let it upset you.

LILY pushes MADELAINE away.

FLORRIE: Well, I have to say he deserved that.

JESSIE: Yes, well done Lily.

ALICE: Come on, we'd better go.

The music and dancing stop and they all exit.

Movement sequence with ALFRED, JACK and HERBERT indicating the first three games against the French. They respond to the scores of the previous three games. The scores are chalked on the board as part of the sequence:

30/04/1920 Dick, Kerr's 2, French xi 0

01/05/1920 Dick, Kerr's 5, French xi 2

05/05/1920 Dick, Kerr's 1, French xi 1

ALFRED/COMMENTARY: After two wins and a draw, it's all eyes on Stamford Bridge.

They exit.

SCENE TWO

Stamford Bridge.

ALICE, FLORRIE and JESSIE enter and are engaged in a pre-match warm-up.

JESSIE: I still can't get used to that hotel.

FLORRIE: That Henry was a cheeky bugger suggesting we don't have hotels or electricity oop north.

JESSIE: He's been showing me some good places though.

FLORRIE: I hope you've got some energy for today. You look done in. I couldn't live in London.

JESSIE: *(Yawning.)* I could. I love it.

ALFRED enters.

ALFRED: Keeping you up, am I? Right, then ladies I don't know what the heck happened in Blackpool to only earn us a draw in Manchester but the sea air obviously did the French some good so I want to see some real effort today.

ALFRED exits.

JESSIE: Why is Pop in a bad mood?

FLORRIE: He got a load of complaints from the hotel manager.

JESSIE: What about?

FLORRIE: Too much noise at night and guests having to wait ages for the bathrooms.

JESSIE: Well what do they expect with baths that size and hot running water at all times?

FLORRIE: Not that you'd know, seeing as you were sneaking off with Henry.

ALICE: I'm not best pleased at having to cover for you.

FLORRIE: I'm not sure Pop believed her either.

JESSIE: Pop's a soft touch.

'La Marseillaise' begins to play and the rest all enter and stand to attention. MADELAINE enters and shakes hands with FLORRIE. ALFRED and JACK take their place on the bench. A stylised game begins.

Sfx: game noise. A goal is scored. Sfx whistle half-time.

JACK: We still need a better goalkeeper.

ALFRED: Aye, I know.

Sfx whistle start game. The stylised game restarts. JESSIE is fouled.

JACK: Bloody hell, that's a foul.

ALFRED: Is that Jessie who's down? It is. She's out cold.

JACK: She's been off her game all afternoon. I'm going on.

JACK and BETTY with a first aid bag run onto the pitch. JACK and BETTY help JESSIE off. FLORRIE follows.

Sfx: whistle (full-time).

HERBERT chalks the score up:

'Dick, Kerr's: 1, French xi: 2'

They all exit apart from ALFRED and MADELAINE.

SCENE THREE

ALFRED: Despite your size, I've been very impressed with your goalkeeping.

MADELAINE: After playing against your team I know I need to improve. They are, how you say, very physical.

ALFRED: How would you like to come back to Preston with us and improve your skills?

MADELAINE: I would like that very much. Merci, monsieur. But I cannot play for you in France.

ALFRED: A shame, but I understand.

MADELAINE exits and LILY, ALICE and FLORRIE enter. MADELAINE smiles at LILY as she exits.

LILY: What's she looking at?

ALFRED: Bad luck, ladies. You acquitted yourselves very well with only ten of you.

FLORRIE: How is Jessie?

ALFRED: She'll be fine. Don't think I don't know what she was getting up to though and that I'm not disappointed. I don't blame any of you for not saying anything. Loyalty is all very well and good but not when it affects the team.

FLORRIE: Sorry, Pop.

ALFRED: You're going to have a chance to have another go. We've been invited over to France later this year…and Madamoiselle Ourry has decided to come back to Preston with us to improve her goalkeeping skills.

LILY: Does that mean we'll have to eat garlic?

They all exit apart from LILY and ALICE. MRS WOODS enters.

SCENE FOUR

MRS WOODS parlour. LILY is standing and ALICE sitting. ALICE has a piece of paper. MRS WOODS has a tape measure. ALICE is writing on the paper.

MRS WOODS: My, Lily, I do hope you've stopped growing. That's five foot ten I make you.

LILY: It's very good of you to help me. I wish I could write like you, Alice. It's so neat and pretty.

ALICE: They want to know a lot don't they? I do hope the food is all right over there.

MRS WOODS: It's all frogs legs and snails.

ALICE: Oh don't say that, Mam. Lily'll be fine – she eats anything.

LILY: I do not.

ALICE: I was only teasing, Lil.

MRS WOODS: Are you sure you don't want to stay for supper, Lily?

LILY: That's very kind of you to ask, Mrs Woods, but I'd best be getting back soon.

MRS WOODS exits.

ALICE: Have you had a word with Florrie yet?

LILY: No. I don't think I've got what it takes.

ALICE: That's nonsense, Lily. You'd make a wonderful nurse.

LILY: I can't read and write like you, Alice. My spelling's rubbish.

ALICE: That doesn't matter. Come on, we'll go through some basics.

LILY: You've always been so kind to me, Alice. You knock off my rough edges.

ALICE: I'm not sure about that. Anyway I think you've given me confidence.

LILY: I have?

ALICE takes hold of LILY's hand briefly.

ALICE: Yes. I love my family and my mam especially of course I do… *(Beat.)* But sometimes I just feel so stifled and the football and people like you make me feel different somehow. Mother would call that swanking but it doesn't feel like it to me.

LILY: I know what you mean. I feel different from other girls too.

LILY takes hold of ALICE's hand and cautiously moves into ALICE as if to kiss her.

ALICE: What are you doing, Lily?

LILY: I thought you liked me, Alice.

ALICE: I do, Lily, but I don't know what you're doing… I don't understand…

LILY lets go of ALICE's hand.

LILY: *(Almost angrily.)* I wasn't doing owt. Anyway I have to go.

She exits.

ALICE: Lily, come back.

ALICE goes after her.

SCENE FIVE

The doors swing open at the factory end and the girls stream in: French flags are on the reverse of the doors. The chalkboard reads: Paris, 1920.

They sing 'The Lasses From Lancashire'.

JESSIE and FLORRIE take in the sights.

JESSIE: So, the great Lily Parr is afraid of heights then?

FLORRIE: She wasn't sick on the ferry over though.

JESSIE: All right. Very funny. Where is she?

FLORRIE: She's gone off with Madelaine somewhere.

JESSIE: What are they going to talk about? I shouldn't think either of them can understand what the other's saying.

FLORRIE: Are you really thinking of moving down to London, Jessie?

JESSIE: Yes. It opened my eyes when we were down there. All the entertainment and there's just so much more going on.

FLORRIE: Not to mention Henry!

JESSIE: I don't know what you mean!

FLORRIE: I can't believe you've kept in touch.

JESSIE: We just seemed to hit it off. Anyway, he's said I can stay with his sister to begin with and he reckons I'll find some work soon enough.

FLORRIE: I have to say I'm enjoying all this travel. Hey up here comes Alice.

ALICE enters.

ALICE: Sorry, I was just talking to some of the French team. They've been teaching me a bit of the language.

JESSIE: I can't understand a word of it.

ALICE: It's hard but I'm picking it up a bit. How about you, Florrie?

FLORRIE: I can understand a little bit.

ALICE: I'm really enjoying it over here.

JESSIE: You are, aren't you?

ALICE: I don't know what it is, but I somehow feel the further away I am from home the more I can just be me. That sounds silly, I know.

JESSIE: No, it doesn't. I think I know how you feel.

ALICE: Still, there's no place like home and I miss my family.

FLORRIE: Will you still play when you and Herbert are married?

ALICE: Well, not when we have a family.

FLORRIE: I wouldn't want to let being married stop me doing what I wanted.

JESSIE: I don't think I would, either.

FLORRIE: You'd better make the most of it, then, Alice as it's not long now till the wedding.

ALICE, FLORRIE and JESSIE exit with the latter two humming the wedding march.

SCENE SIX

Paris, 1920s French flags on the doors. LILY and MADELAINE enter.

MADELAINE: I did not expect you English ladies to be so how you say on the field?

LILY: Rough?

MADELAINE: Rough. That means physical?

LILY: Yes.

MADELAINE: But off the field you are…

LILY: Still rough?

MADELAINE: No. I think you could be if you tried more – be an elegant lady.

LILY: I've never been called elegant before. *(Beat.)* I wasn't sure I'd cope out in France.

MADELAINE: Are we so different?

LILY: People reckon I am.

MADELAINE: Maybe I will come back again to Preston one day. Would you like that?

LILY: I don't know. I suppose so. Now that I know you better.

MADELAINE: And you no longer think I am arrogant French lady?

LILY: I never thought that.

MADELAINE: I will miss you, Lily. You are, a very intriguing lady.

LILY: Get away with you.

MADELAINE: I wish you could stay here longer.

LILY: I have a hard time making mesen understood in English.

MADELAINE: But you will meet someone. Someone like you. Adieu.

LILY: Goodbye.

LILY offers her hand to shake but MADELAINE clasps LILY to her and hugs her then kisses her. LILY starts to pull away.

MADELAINE: Ne t'inquiète pas. On fait pas de mal, Lily.

MADELAINE kisses LILY again. LILY begins to exit but forgets her bag in the moment, and MADELAINE calls her back for it.

MADELAINE: Your valise Lily.

LILY: Cheers.

MADELINE exits through the doors. Doors close. LILY exits at the domestic end.

SCENE SEVEN

Repeated movement sequence with ALFRED, JACK and HERBERT of some matches when Dick, Kerr's Ladies are achieving increasingly good gates and results from 1921. Scores are chalked up on the board or projected:

Dick, Kerr's 8, St Helen's 1

Dick, Kerr's 10, Rest of Lancashire 0

Dick Kerr's 8, Ellesmere Port 0

Sfx: football crowds.

As the sequence ends, JACK and HERBERT set the benches to recreate the bar.

FLORRIE and JESSIE enter. FLORRIE has a 'Football Bits' magazine, JESSIE has a small case.

FLORRIE: Have you seen this?

JESSIE: What is it?

FLORRIE: It's that new magazine 'Football Bits'. Someone calling themselves 'Football Girl' reckons Dick, Kerr's are not as good as they used to be and because we win easily we don't try as hard.

JESSIE: That don't make sense.

FLORRIE: There's another article written by some doctor or other saying that playing football is harmful to the female form. They may receive injuries from which they may never recover.

JESSIE: I'd like to see that doctor do a day's work at a factory.

ALFRED enters with JACK.

ALFRED: It's been a pleasure, Jessie.

JESSIE: Thank you Pop. I've had a wonderful time.

FLORRIE: You make sure he treats you right.

JESSIE: I will, don't you worry.

FLORRIE: Give him a good kick you know where if he don't.

JESSIE: I will.

FLORRIE: Hope you have a good life, Jessie. I'll miss you.

JESSIE: I'll miss you too.

FLORRIE: Don't forget where you came from though. We don't want you going soft down there.

JESSIE: There's no chance of that.

ALICE enters.

ALICE: I was worried I'd missed you!

JESSIE: No, I'm getting the train this afternoon. I'm going to make some sandwiches and everything!

FLORRIE: Well, come on then, I'll walk with you to the end of the street.

FLORRIE and JESSIE exit, arm in arm.

ALFRED: What can I do for you, Mrs Stanley?

ALICE: Oh, Pop – I don't think I'll ever get used to not being Alice Woods!!

ALFRED: What did you want to see me about, Alice?

ALICE: Well, it's a couple of things, but I'll wait for Lily to get here to tell you about one of them.

ALFRED: So, what's the first thing?

ALICE: It's about Lily.

ALFRED: What about her?

ALICE: I don't think she's very happy.

ALFRED: What makes you say that?

ALICE: She's always so moody.

ALFRED: That's just Lily.

ALICE: But even more so lately. She only seems happy when she's on the field. I don't think factory work suits her. I've seen her with men wounded in the war – men like Len – and she really helps them.

ALFRED: I think you're right, there. Lord knows, she's never on time and her mind always seems to be elsewhere. There may be a way I can help.

LILY enters.

ALFRED: Now then, Lily – what's on your mind?

LILY: We want to see if we can play some games to help the striking miners.

ALFRED: Oh yes?

LILY: We're St Helens girls, me and Alice. We look after our own. People are starving all cos of this bloody government.

ALICE: We have to help them. They've already had their wages docked in half and now they're locked out.

ALFRED: Yes I know, it's a terrible business. Leave it with me and I'll do my best for you, I promise.

ALFRED and JACK go over to bar. ALICE winces noticeably.

LILY: Are you all right, Alice?

ALICE: It's nothing. Just a pain I get from time to time.

LILY: How long have you had it?

ALICE: A few months now.

LILY: You've never said.

ALICE: Because it's nothing. I feel fine now. Come on Lily.

Something in ALICE's expression suggests that this has been more than the usual pain. They exit.

ALFRED and JACK move from the bar.

JACK: I don't think it's a good idea at all, Alf. Playing matches for striking miners.

ALFRED: Why not?

JACK: The FA have tolerated us whilst we raised money for injured servicemen but they are not going to like this.

ALFRED: The FA are a bunch of stuck-up self-righteous prigs. Those girls are right. People are starving.

JACK: I know they are, but I'm not sure this is the right way to help them.

ALFRED: I can't understand why the FA have objected to us having a meal when we played away. The men's players do it.

JACK: You don't have to tell me.

ALFRED: We've got nothing to hide.

JACK: We've shown how easy it is to make money out of the game. That's what they don't like.

ALFRED: They don't want people asking where the money in men's football goes.

JACK: And you're sure you can account for all of ours?

ALFRED: We covered our expenses no more, no less and raised thousands for charity.

JACK: Yes, charity for injured servicemen. Nobody's going to argue about that. But miner's on strike?

ALFRED: But look at the publicity Dick, Kerr's received.

JACK: Yes, and some of the board were far from happy with that publicity. And playing matches for striking miners is only going to antagonise the rest of the board that you haven't already.

ALFRED: Well, most of them can't see the wood for the trees. You know what it means to those girls to be playing football.

JACK: That's all well and good but the tide is turning Alf. We're the victims of our own success.

ALFRED: What does that mean? We've been too successful? That doesn't make sense to me.

JACK: The backlash is starting. Don't burn all your bridges though.

ALFRED: Oh I know where my loyalties lie.

They exit and the bar is struck.

SCENE EIGHT

MRS WOODS at the parlour domestic end of the set. Armchair is set.

MRS WOODS enters, followed by MRS PARR.

MRS PARR sits on the edge of the seat of the armchair.

MRS WOODS: It must be nice having Lily home for a couple of days.

MRS PARR: Yes, although she's moaning about having to share a room again.

MRS WOODS: I've kept Alice's room just the same as when she was here. It seems strange to think she's a married woman now – I don't know where the time goes.

MRS PARR: Doesn't seem five minutes since they started playing for Dick, Kerr's. It's been the making of our Lily.

MRS WOODS: It's a shame you can't go to the match, though. It looks like I was lucky to get a ticket

MRS PARR: My men folk are out on strike.

MRS WOODS: I know, it must be hard.

MRS PARR: It didn't help that the railway workers wouldn't strike as well.

MRS WOODS: I've got relatives who work on the railways. Why should they go on strike? The miners could have tried harder to make a deal.

MRS PARR: I'm not going to argue with you.

MRS WOODS: I'm sorry. It's not your fault.

MRS PARR: At least the football matches are raising some money for us.

MRS WOODS: Well, I'm not sure that I agree with the strike or girls playing football for that matter although I suppose I can see the good it can do.

MRS PARR: At least you get to see your girl play.

They exit.

SCENE NINE

Set up for Goodison Park: the chalkboard is written on with the teams – Dick, Kerr's Ladies vs St Helens and the date – 26 december 1920.

ALFRED and JACK enter surveying the pitch.

ALFRED: Look at that, Jack – they reckon there's close to 53,000 people here today.

JACK: The groundsman said his son plays for the boy's team here and they're lucky to get a quarter of the support Dick, Kerr's do.

ALFRED: The FA are still getting complaints about people making money out of these charity matches.

JACK: It's who we're raising money for. I did try to warn you. The FA won't want to be getting involved with the trade unions.

ALFRED: We've all got to look out for each other. Why shouldn't we help people along the way?

JACK: It's all got too political – in lots of ways: the men's clubs have started complaining that their games are being overshadowed, and other teams are saying that our matches are all one-sided now as we've pinched all the best players going.

ALFRED: What? That's nonsense. Absolute nonsense.

ALICE and LILY enter.

ALICE: Alf, Alf – Florrie's missed her train.

ALFRED: What? That's all we need on our biggest ever game.

The ladies come back on stage and a choreographed game without a ball begins.

LILY gives Dick, Kerr's a 1-0 lead.

Sfx: whistle for half-time.

ALFRED: We're doing all right, ladies but we've only got a one nil lead. Alice *(looking at ALICE)* I want you to play centre forward. Show their goalkeeper a bit more menace, all right?

ALICE: Yes. Come on you lot let's show them what Dick, Kerr's girls are made of.

LADIES: Yes Alice.

During the second half ALICE scores a hat-trick. Chalkboard is updated:

Dick, Kerr's 4, St Helens 0

The final whistle. ALICE is doubled over, seemingly at the effort of the match. LILY approaches her –

LILY: I don't believe you Alice Wood. First time at centre
forward and you score a hat-trick. Wait a minute! That
means that you get to keep the match ball.

LILY runs across the stage.

Oi yous give us that ball back unless you want a good
thumping.

ALICE groans in pain.

Are you all right, Alice? Oh God, someone get a doctor
quick.

*ALICE is supported in the centre circle by JACK and the actress
playing BETTY.*

SCENE TEN

*Two doctors enter (white coats/stethoscopes/clipboards) followed by
other members of the team also in white coats. They begin to walk the
corridors busily. MRS WOODS and HERBERT look on anxiously trying
to get them to answer their questions.*

ALFRED: 'We can in no way sanction the reckless exposure
to violence of organs which the common experience of
women has led them in every way to protect.'

HERBERT: Excuse me –

LEN: 'The kicking is too jerky a movement for women, and
the strain is likely to be severe.'

MRS WOODS: I'm looking for Alice Stanley – she's my
daughter –

ALFRED: 'Should they get similar knocks and buffetings their
future duties as mothers would be seriously impaired...'

HERBERT: Excuse me –

FLORRIE: 'They may receive injuries from which they may never recover...'

MRS WOODS: I'm looking for Alice Stanley – she's my daughter –

JESSIE: 'There are physical reasons why the game is harmful to women...'

DOCTOR 2: 'It is a rough game at any time, but it is much more harmful to women than men...'

HERBERT: Excuse me –

LILY: 'A most unsuitable game: too much for a woman's physical frame.'

MRS WOODS/HERBERT: Excuse me –

The opinions build until they are distorted – ALICE is bewildered in the centre.

HERBERT: *(Shouting.)* Will someone just tell me what is going on!

The space clears and they all exit leaving HERBERT and MRS WOODS standing together.

MRS WOODS: But it can't be good for her playing rough sports.

HERBERT: She's been fine until now...

MRS WOODS: And now she's expecting. I thought once you were married she'd stop playing so much football.

HERBERT: Sport is important to her. It's part of who she is.

The DOCTOR enters.

MRS WOODS: Doctor, how is she? How is the baby? Will it be damaged?

DOCTOR: No, not at all.

MRS WOODS: You are sure about that?

DOCTOR: Mrs Woods I have known women do all kinds of
    hard work before and during the war whilst expecting and
    still have perfectly healthy babies... If you'd like to follow
    me, I'll take you to see her.

They exit.

ALFRED and JACK enter.

ALFRED: So, we're settled then – I'll go to London and
    present all our evidence to the meeting at the Football
    Association. The statement from the lady doctor saying
    how women playing football is perfectly healthy and safe,
    and the accounts to show that everything's above board
    and the money has been going to the charities we say it's
    been going to.

JACK: Best of luck, Alfred

They shake hands. They exit.

SCENE 11

*The girls are all together in the pub – FLORRIE is going to canada, and
this is her leaving party. ALICE and HERBERT, LILY, FLORRIE, JACK,
BETTY and DAISY enter. There is a light atmosphere: general pub noise
underscores. JACK and HERBERT seem preoccupied.*

DAISY: So, are you all packed, Florrie?

FLORRIE: I've only got to take a few things on the boat, and
    then I can send for the rest when I'm settled.

BETTY: It's quite an adventure you're going on.

FLORRIE: It's a new start.

LILY: I can't see what there is there that you can't get here.

FLORRIE: More opportunities, wider skies, Lily – it's time you broadened your horizons. There's more jobs for nurses like you and me out there. You should think about it.

LILY: I'm happy where I am, thanks.

DAISY: But it's such a long way!

FLORRIE: I know Daisy – that's the only thing I'm worried about. Who's going to be just round the corner when I'm thousands of miles away?

ALICE: Seems like there are changes in store for all of us.

BETTY: Do you remember when I sometimes missed the start of our kickabouts?

FLORRIE: You had your reasons – we know that now.

DAISY: Jack, where's Pop? He's not usually late.

JACK: I'll go to the end of the street and see if I can see him.

HERBERT: I'll come an'all – I could do with a stroll.

HERBERT and JACK get up to leave. As they begin to exit ALFRED meets them at the door. He appears sombre and tired. He gives a folder of papers to HERBERT.

JACK: Here he is! Come on Alfred, let me get you a drink – looks like you could do with one.

ALFRED takes off his coat and places his hat on the table. HERBERT and JACK look at the papers.

LILY: Come on, Pop – you look like you've lost half a crown and found a farthing! We're celebrating getting rid of Florrie and having me as the new team captain!

FLORRIE: Now that's a good enough reason to make me change my mind!!

ALFRED: There'll be no more football.

DAISY: No, we're still going to play when she's gone – we've got the home match at Deepdale next week, and then –

ALFRED: We'll not be playing at Deepdale next week Daisy, or any other week from now on.

LILY: What – why not?

ALFRED: I've been to a meeting of the Football Association in London – not that they let me speak – and the FA have decided that we can't play at Deepdale or at any other FA affiliated grounds anymore.

DAISY: Why have they singled us out?

ALICE: Just Dick, Kerr's Ladies?

ALFRED: No, all women's football teams – not just you.

FLORRIE: So they've effectively banned us from playing?

BETTY: That's just spiteful!

ALFRED: They believe football is quite unsuitable for the female form and it shouldn't be encouraged.

ALICE: That's what they said?

ALFRED: They wouldn't hear the evidence of the doctor I found.

HERBERT: They've said that the women's game is full of financial irregularities

ALICE: Like what?

HERBERT consults some notes.

HERBERT: They claimed an excessive proportion of the receipts are absorbed in expenses and an 'inadequate percentage' devoted to charitable objects.

ALICE: Is that true?

HERBERT: Of course not. We've raised thousands for charity.

JACK: I reckon it was playing matches for the miners that did it for us.

ALFRED: They threw everything they could at us.

FLORRIE: What's wrong with raising money to help people?

ALFRED: Nothing except when it's for striking miners.

FLORRIE: And the money went to the miners?

ALFRED: Of course it did.

LILY: You promised you'd look after us.

ALICE: I can't help thinking it's our fault. If Lily and I hadn't suggested it in the first place –

A beat as they take it in.

JACK: I'd like to say summat. Ladies, when I agreed to come and be your trainer I thought I'd be a laughing stock but I've come to see that you've got as much dedication, passion and skill as any in the men's game. You can all be very proud of what you've achieved. I'm going to miss coaching you.

LILY: They can't stop us playing on the recreation grounds though, can they? People would still come and watch.

JACK: No they can't, as long as it's not an FA ground where the men's matches are played.

FLORRIE: Why not go on tour? Come to Canada maybe?

ALICE: Couldn't there be a ladie's league? Along the lines of the men's game?

ALFRED: We'll find a way to carry on somehow. We'll play on ploughed fields if we have to. This team will go on.

LILY: Sod the FA.

ALL: Sod the FA.

ALICE: To Dick, Kerr's Ladies.

ALL: To Dick, Kerr's Ladies.

JACK has moved away from the main group. Whilst everyone else exits LILY goes over to him.

LILY: Are you going to stay with us Jack?

JACK doesn't reply. He gives her his empty glass. LILY touches him on the shoulder.

Goodnight Jack.

He exits. The furniture is cleared. LILY follows where ALFRED left.

SCENE ELEVEN

ALFRED enters by a street lamp followed by LILY, catching up with him near the factory.

LILY: Pop, wait – I can't help thinking it's all my fault.

ALFRED: How can you think that?

LILY: If we hadn't asked you to play matches for the miners.

ALFRED: You only asked. I made the decision and I'd do the same again.

LILY: Then there's all the, the…

ALFRED: The what, Lily?

LILY: Nasty talk about ladie's teams being full of, of dirty practices.

ALFRED: And not your tackling! It's all right. None of it is your fault.

LILY: It's just so wrong though.

ALFRED: Aye, it is. Don't you worry though.
I'll make sure you're all right.

LILY: You're a good man, Pop.

ALFRED: You know what managing this team has taught me Lily?

LILY shakes her head.

There's nothing that women shouldn't be allowed to do that men can. Never stop believing that, Lily.

They embrace then ALFRED exits.

SCENE TWELVE

FLORRIE enters.

LILY: So you're all set to go, then?

FLORRIE: I am, yes.

LILY: It's a big step.

FLORRIE: I know, but I'm looking forward to it.

LILY: I couldn't leave here.

FLORRIE: I can't stay here. I need to be somewhere that's… oh I don't know… I just need to be somewhere else.

LILY: Well, Pop's still organising games for us – the crowds won't be so big – but at least we're still playing football.

FLORRIE: It's not the same as it was though, is it? It never will be.

LILY: No, you're right, it's not – but it won't be forever.

FLORRIE: I need to get away and try something new before it's too late. Anyway, are you coming? Pop said that goalkeeper chap were meeting us at one. Bloody cheek, saying you couldn't put one past him!

LILY: I'll catch you up!

FLORRIE exits as ALICE enters.

Hello, stranger – where've you been hiding? I've missed you.

ALICE: Well, we've been a bit busy getting ready for the baby coming.

LILY: That's ages yet. You really didn't know you were pregnant?

ALICE: No.

LILY: Where's Herbert?

ALICE: Gone to speak to Pop. I think he misses working for him.

LILY: We could do with you back on the team.

ALICE: I think my football days are over Lily. Are you still enjoying it?

LILY: Yes, but I miss playing in front of a big crowd.

ALICE: Still, we showed them all eh? Women can play football.

LILY: I think we scared 'em all.

ALICE: How do you mean?

LILY: Most men want it to go back to how it was before the war, and before the vote was granted, women staying at home and having babies. Not that you and Herbert are like that though.

ALICE: It's all right Lily. How's it going at the Whittingham?

LILY: I'm enjoying it. I've made a new friend.

ALICE: That's good. What's her name?

LILY: Mary. How'd you know it was a woman?

ALICE: Come on Lily. I'm not that naive any more. I hope you are happy.

LILY: Aye I am. Happiest I've ever been.

FLORRIE enters with ALFRED, HERBERT and FRED.

FLORRIE: Here he is!

ALFRED: I'd like you to meet Fred. As you know, he's a professional keeper who doesn't think Lily's capable of putting a shot past him.

FRED: Aye, I've heard all about you. You might look good against other lassies but you'd be no match for a proper professional player

LILY: You look familiar. Are you sure we haven't met before?

FRED: You'd definitely remember if we had!

He makes his trademark gesture of ducking and diving which reminds LILY where she has seen him before.

There are shouts of 'You show him Lily' as they set themselves up near a goal.

FRED: Give it your best shot, love!

LILY: This one's for you, Alice.

With a minimal run up LILY smashes an imaginary ball at FRED. He puts his arm out to stop it but the force of the shot propels him into the goal.

FRED: Bloody hell, she's broke me bloody arm!.

ALFRED walks over to FRED and helps him off stage. ALFRED is struggling not to laugh. All the girls congratulate LILY and lift her onto their shoulders as they carry her out.

ALICE returns, dressed as she was as the beginning of the play. She is carrying the leather football and a pair of boots. She places the boots just behind the centre spot – facing the factory end. The cast begin to hum 'Abide with Me' from off stage to underscore ALICE's speech.

LILY in her football kit comes through the factory gates and stands where her portrait was at the start.

She and ALICE are facing each other.

ALICE: I remember it all, Lily... What a time it was. We may have played for a Preston team but your heart was always here in St Helens…and you kept playing even though the FA ban lasted for fifty years… You've been a real inspiration to any young lass who thinks she can't do something because of her gender.

She places the ball on the centre spot.

Near on a thousand goals you scored in your career, Lil! Now that's a record – aren't many chaps who have rivalled that!

Bless you, Lily Parr, you had a heart of gold and a kick strong enough to crack a crossbar, and break a man's arm!

Well, Lil, I hope you're giving the angels grief with some hard cussing and hard tackling.

The cast enter singing and building 'Abide with Me' in a rousing chorus then exit. At the same time the lights gradually fade until a single spot picks out LILY's boots and the ball.

Sfx: – final whistle.

Full time.

WWW.OBERONBOOKS.COM

Follow us on www.twitter.com/@oberonbooks
& www.facebook.com/OberonBooksLondon